One Month to Neuromuscular Health

Felicia Assenza, Jalee Pelissier, Pauline Nichol

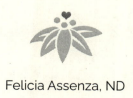

Felicia Assenza, ND

Copyright © 2022 FELICIA ASSENZA. All rights reserved.

Published by FELICIA ASSENZA, ND

ISBN 978-1-387-95275-5

Contents

Dedication — V

Introduction — VI
    What is Neuromuscular Health?
    Why This Program?
    Materials Needed
    Reaching out for Help

My Story — IX

1. Mindset — 1
    Day 1: Brain DUMP
    Day 2: Gratitude
    Day 3: Letter to your body
    Day 4: If I was "normal", I would...
    Day 5: What if there is no such thing as normal?
    Day 6: Let's get grounded
    Day 7: Time to set those intentions

2. Nutrition   7
    Day 1: The food journal
    Day 2: Protein
    Day 3: Fruits and veggies
    Day 4: Grains, breads, and starches
    Day 5: Healthy fats
    Day 6: Whole foods for whole bodies
    Day 7: The grocery shop

Food Journal Template   16

3. Exercise   17
    Day 1: Range of motion
    Day 2: Stretch it out
    Day 3: Really stretch it out
    Day 4: Building strength
    Day 5: Sweat it out
    Day 6: How do you like to move?
    Day 7: Putting it all together

4. Connection   31
    Day 1: Who's in your corner?
    Day 2: Whose corner are you in?
    Day 3: Communities
    Day 4: Connecting to something bigger
    Day 5: Revisiting intentions
    Day 6: Bringing intentions to life
    Day 7: Wrap-up

Complementary Care Resource Network   36

Acknowledgments   37

Author and Contributors   38

One Month to Neuromuscular Health is dedicated to all of those willing to work on their health and learn along the way. Ten percent of the proceeds from this book will be donated to Muscular Dystrophy Canada, the organization that inspired the idea in me that I could use my own challenging health experiences to help make the path a little easier for others.

Introduction

What is Neuromuscular Health?

Neuromuscular health refers to two major body systems, the nervous system and the muscular system and how the two interact to keep the body moving well. It is my goal with this program to keep things practical so I am going to refrain from delving too deep into the theoretical aspects of the neuromuscular system and leave that to the neurologists. I will say though that it is fascinating to learn the inner workings and interactions of both these systems and would highly encourage further reading on the neuromuscular system if you have the chance!

Studying the inner workings of these two systems specifically can help us learn about them and how to best support them. However, when it comes to health - including neuromuscular health - I believe it is important to look at the whole person. In my naturopathic practice and in my own personal experience, neuromuscular health becomes less about the neurons (cells of the nervous system) and muscle fibres that keep us moving and more about:
- How we move
- How we want to move

INTRODUCTION

- Why we want to move
- How we best support the nervous and muscular systems and all of our other body systems to keep us moving

I also want to take a moment to talk about movement and what that looks like. I want to highlight the importance of recognizing that movement looks different for everyone and even looks different for the same person on different days or at different points in time. Observing your movement without judgement is a great way to start getting familiar with your body and how you move. This is something we will talk about at length throughout the program.

Why This Program?

My experience with neuromuscular disease (NMD) led to a career in healthcare so that I could help make the path a little easier for others with unique abilities. The aim of this program is to give you an introduction to a new way of approaching muscle health. Please realize, this program is not a quick fix or four-week magic cure.

Instead, the program is designed to empower you to take your health into your own hands and change your perspective. This month is more like a starting point, a roadmap if you will, to figure out what you really want out of life and how to get there. The driving or how you get there is always up to you. It is my hope that by the end of these four weeks you will have a new way of looking at neuromuscular health, maybe even health in general, and feel inspired to live your very best life.

You will also notice that this program does not only address physical health. It is my firm belief that optimal health involves a beautiful balance of the mind, body, and spirit. As such, this course incorporates working on all three areas of health and bringing them together in harmony.

Materials Needed

All you will need is a journal, a pen (or device to type or audio/video record), a highlighter, some space to move, an open mind, and 30 minutes each day.

Reaching out for Help

While there is a lot of talk about taking health into your own hands, that does not mean tackling your health challenges all on your own. We all need help. In fact, many of us do our best when we have support. You may even find it helpful to do this program with a family member or friend. We could all benefit from working on our neuromuscular health, NMD or not. You could even try joining the One Month to Neuromuscular Health Facebook support group for the book, where you can connect with people who have completed or are currently working through the program.

We'll also be talking about some pretty big things here. If you are struggling with getting started, staying on track, or need some extra support at any point in the program, please reach out for help. You can even refer to our growing network of Ontario providers who are familiar with neuromuscular health here or at the end of this book.

My Story

Not long after my birth, it became apparent to my parents that something was different. I did not flop like other babies did and my muscles seemed tighter and more stiff. My mother often says that with my tight shoulders and balled up fists, I looked like I was ready for a fight. After a few confusing appointments with a pediatrician, then an orthopedic specialist, I ended up having my first (and only) surgery at 6 months, a hip adductor tenotomy for those who like fancy medical jargon. It basically means I had a tendon cut in my hips to relieve tension and spent the next few months in an orthotic brace. That was the start of 18 years of what I lovingly call, specialist hopping.

My wonderful, loving parents took me from specialist to specialist where there was always a lot of head scratching, diagnostic tests, caring health professionals, and more questions than answers. At 18 years old, when I finally received a diagnosis that stuck, I think my neuromuscular specialist who had been scratching his head for years was more excited than I was. If you have ever seen the cartoon image of the stick person jumping for joy and clicking his heels together, this is the image I have in my head of my neuromuscular specialist on that day. More than 10 years after that, my diagnosis has again changed but I have come to realize that a diagnosis is not all that important anyway.

What sometimes comes as a surprise to those I tell my story to is when I say that not having a real diagnosis for 18 years was a ginormous blessing. You see, in all my years of specialist hopping, I had the opportunity to interact with some pretty incredible people. I had the opportunity to watch problem solving at work in some of the brightest minds. I learned that, sometimes, simple caring and reassurance did more for my healing than the newest, most technologically advanced diagnostic testing. I learned what it meant to be a patient and it was here that I was first inspired to one day be on the other end. I just needed a couple more experiences to help me decide exactly how I wanted to be on the other end and what sort of healthcare provider I wanted to be.

It was not until my second year in university that I started to realize, while there were lots of options out there to help me in my healing, my healing was ultimately my responsibility. This realization, that my health was in my hands, led me to seek out more empowering styles of medicine, ones where I learned how to understand my body, my needs, and how to meet them. This realization would eventually lead me to the study of naturopathic medicine. I fell in love with the holistic approach to health and am proud to say that I am now a practicing Naturopathic Doctor. While it still came with many challenges along the way, I do not think I could have dreamed of a better career for myself and am beyond honoured that I have the privilege of working with people and being a part of their health journeys while continuing to pursue my own.

Mindset

When it comes to neuromuscular health, we tend to look at things from a physical angle. If you have ever tried to work on your neuromuscular health, it is likely that you have thought about how much you want to lift, how far you want to walk, or what stretches might be best. It is less likely that you have thought about why you want to lift, where you want to walk and why, or what motivates you to stretch.

While looking at the physical aspect is valuable, your motivation and sense of purpose is just as important. Have you ever tried to follow an exercise program that you dreaded doing? How did that go for you? In my experience, an exercise program is usually most helpful and effective if you are motivated to follow it. I find that one of the best motivators is enjoyment. I know I am much more likely to do something that I actually enjoy doing.

The first step in coming up with an exercise program you enjoy is to really figure out what you enjoy and why. That is what we will be doing this week: finding our why or what brings us joy, fulfillment and purpose. From there we will come up with goals and intentions that will be the basis for a work-out plan and lifestyle change that we actually enjoy. If you would like to learn more about finding your purpose, Simon Sinek, author of *Find Your Why*, has a few great books to help including *Start with Why* and *Find your Why*[1]. Now without further ado, let's jump in!

Day 1: Brain DUMP

I always find it nice to clear my mind before starting something new. Anyone else have trouble clearing their head? Today's exercise is one that is particularly helpful for getting all of those thoughts out of your head and onto paper. You may even be surprised at what comes out of that beautiful brain of yours. This is a great exercise to do anytime, especially when you are feeling overwhelmed by your thoughts, having trouble quieting your mind, or even when you need to make a difficult decision. This is how it works:
1. Pull out your journal.
2. Take note of how you are feeling before this activity.
3. Set a timer for two minutes. You can try even longer if you are feeling adventurous.
4. Write down anything that comes to mind. Write down any frustrations, grievances, joys, things that you are thankful for, etc. Anything that comes to mind is relevant. The only rule is that the pen does not leave the page for the full two minutes. If you cannot think of anything, write about that. It could look something like... "Nothing comes to mind, I don't like this activity..." Anything goes, just keep writing for at least two minutes.
5. Take note of how you are feeling after this activity. Were there any changes?

Day 2: Gratitude

What are you thankful for? It can sometimes be a little too easy to get so caught up in what we do not have or what we cannot do that we lose sight of what we do have and what we can do. My earliest memory of learning about gratitude came from the classic book *Pollyanna* by Eleanor Porter, "... there is something about everything that you can be glad about, if you keep hunting long enough to find it."[2] Modern research seems to agree with Pollyanna here. The more people express their gratitude or thanks for what they do have in their lives, the happier they are and the easier it is to make positive changes in their lives[3]. Over time, the more you start to pay attention to what you do have in your life the easier it becomes to focus on the positive attributes of your life.

In today's task, we are writing down what we are thankful for. The goal is to come up with a list of at least ten things. If you have never done something like this before or if you struggle with depression or low moods, this can be quite challenging. Do your best and know that it does get easier with practice. Also remember that there is nothing too small to be thankful for. Sometimes my gratitude lists include things like clean air, water, the sun, the rain; anything that you feel grateful for counts!

Day 3: Letter to your body

Our bodies also talk to us in many ways. One way, for example, is through pain. Pain is our body's way of telling us that something is not quite right. Have you ever talked back to your body? Do you speak to your body with kindness? What would a conversation with your body look like? After living with your body your whole life, maybe it is time to pay attention to your relationship with it. One great way to do this is to write a letter.

It may feel a little strange but I encourage you to try it out. You can tell your body what you are frustrated or sad about, tell it what you are grateful for, ask it what you need to ask it. How the conversation goes is really up to you. If you need a little help to start the conversation, you may want to try something like this: "Dear body, we've been together a while and here are some things I'd like you to know..."

Day 4: If I was "normal", I would...

I find it incredible how many of us think we are not normal. We are all unique individuals so it makes sense that we have some differences. How boring would the world be if we were all the same? One thing I find many of us have in common though is the worry that we are not normal or something is wrong with us. What is normal? Is there a clear definition? How do you define it? Is it being free of disease or disorder? What would you do if you were "normal"?

Sometimes we spend so much time trying to fit in or trying to "be normal" that we forget to actually pay attention to what we really want in life or why we wanted to "be normal" in the first place. Take some time now to visualize what your best life would look like. Take your time with this. You can write about it in your journal or even draw a picture to help you visualize your ideal life.

Day 5: What if there is no such thing as normal?

Reflect on yesterday's activity. What is stopping you from bringing this vision to life? Is there any part of your vision that you can work on right now? Is there a way you can modify the ideas in your vision so that you are still living the life you want to live?

Write the answers to the above questions in your journal.

Take one step today to help you bring your vision to life.

This is where it can be super helpful to work with someone else or a group. You can even join the Facebook support group mentioned at the beginning of the book. Sometimes we can get too fixated on the idea that we need to be "normal" or a certain type of person to be able to live the lives we want. Bringing in another person's perspective can help us see how that is usually not the case. If you are having trouble figuring out how to bring your vision to life, ask for help. A new perspective may open the door to something you did not think was possible.

Day 6: Let's get grounded

Do you have any spiritual practices? Maybe a morning prayer time or daily meditation? Maybe it is spending time in nature? What makes you feel calm, inspired, and at peace? Having a regular spiritual practice has been associated with living longer, coping better, and improved management of stress and illness[4]. It appears that when we have a way to understand the meaning behind suffering, the suffering becomes easier to bear. Spiritual practices help us understand the meaning.

Today's task involves taking five to fifteen minutes to do what makes you feel calm, inspired, and at peace. I have included a short guided meditation below if you need a place to start. My suggestion would be to read through the meditation first, maybe light a candle or play some music if that brings you peace, then close your eyes and try to go by heart.

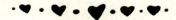

Guided Meditation
In a seated position with both feet on the floor, close your eyes and pay attention to how you are feeling. Notice any sensations, thoughts, or emotions that might pop up.

Pay attention to your breath. Notice if it is fast or slow, deep or shallow. Take three intentional deep breaths. On every breath in, breathe in calm and peace. On every breath out, breathe out tension or anything you want to let go of.

Pay attention to the space between your eyebrows. Notice how it feels. Notice if the muscles in that area are relaxed or tense. See if you can let go of any tension in this area.

Now pay attention to your chest. You can even place your hands over your heart. Imagine a warm pink light in the centre of your chest. Imagine it spreading over your entire body, starting in the chest, then spreading all the way to the top of your head and the tips of your toes. Take a moment to sit in the warm pink light and notice how you are feeling.

When you are ready, let the light return back to your chest and open your eyes ready to make the most of the rest of your day.

Day 7: Time to set those intentions

Okay, now is the time to start turning your vision from Day 4 into a reality. Before putting pen to paper, it would be helpful to first get grounded. Refer to yesterday's lesson and start with a brief meditation or prayer to get you feeling connected, calm, peaceful, and inspired.

Take out your journal and write down anything that comes to mind when you think about what you want to accomplish in life. No limits, just write them down.

Now, pick one to five intentions you would like to work on. For each intention, close your eyes and imagine as vividly as you can what it will be like when this intention becomes a reality. Imagine what it will look like, what it will feel like, who will be around, etc.

List the steps you will take to help you bring this intention to reality. Share this intention with a friend who will hold you accountable. Take your first step to bringing this intention to life today.

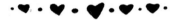

A breath of fresh air: Did you know paying attention to your breathing and taking a couple of deep breaths in and out are great ways to get grounded and bring yourself to the present moment?

---

1. Sinek S. Start with Why. Harlow: Penguin Books; 2011.
2. Porter EH. Pollyanna. United States: L.C. Page; 1913.
3. Publishing HH. Giving thanks can make you happier [Internet]. Health Beat. 2021. Available from: https://www.health.harvard.edu/healthbeat/giving-thanks-can-make-you-happier
4. Puchalski CM. The Role of Spirituality in Health Care. Baylor Univ Med Cent Proc [Internet]. 2001 Oct 1;14(4):352–7. Available from: https://doi.org/10.1080/08998280.2001.11927788

Nutrition

Nutrition is your fuel and, like a car without good fuel, it is difficult to go very far without. Nutrition is a big topic so for the purposes of this program we are going to take a broad, holistic approach. Once you have the basics down, you can dive deeper into the details with your Naturopathic Doctor or Nutritionist.

Wisdom Bite 1: Did you know that if your body does not have enough fuel (glucose), it will start breaking down your fat and muscle tissues for energy?

Wisdom Bite 2: Remember how we talked about enjoyment being a great motivator? This concept applies to nutrition too. The best nutrition involves good food in good company. If you are finding eating good food to be stressful as opposed to fun and enjoyable, check in with someone, it may be time to make some sustainable changes to your daily eating habits.

Please note that this week is a little more involved than last week and can be overwhelming especially if you are someone who may have a complicated relationship with food, body image, or dieting. If you are finding this week overwhelming, take things one day at a time, reach out for help, connect with the Facebook support group, and feel free to space this out to two weeks if needed.

Day 1: The food journal

The food journal is a good way to get a snapshot of what you are eating on a daily basis. Try to leave any judgement out of this process. Simply observe and record what you are eating for one week. This will give you a good idea of whether or not you want to make changes to your diet and where. There is a template at the end of this chapter to use if you would like or you could design your own. It is helpful to include:
- What you are eating
- The portion size
- What time you are eating
- Drinks including water, juice, coffee, tea, alcohol, pop
- Notes on how you are feeling each day

> **Wisdom Bite 3**: It is important to stay hydrated. Each person has different needs when it comes to hydration. Pay attention to your thirst. Have water readily available and when you feel thirsty, drink it.

Day 2: Protein

As we go through this week we will be talking about macronutrients and micronutrients, which can be viewed as large and small nutrients. Protein would fall into the macronutrient category along with carbohydrates and fats. Micronutrients are your vitamins and minerals.

If you have had any experience with trying to build muscle mass, you have probably heard about the importance of protein. The body breaks protein down into amino acids, which are used for various important processes throughout the body. As I mentioned in our first Wisdom Bite of the week, if the body does not get enough fuel it looks for other sources. In this case, if the body needs amino acids it will start breaking down muscle tissue to get them. This is not so great for someone who is trying to build muscle. You may be able to see why having enough protein in your diet can help maintain and build muscle, especially if you are combining it with strength-training exercises[1]. We will talk more about these exercises in Week 3.

Today's task is to include protein with every meal. See if you can fill one third of each plate with foods that are high in protein.

> **Wisdom Bite 4**: Please be aware that eating meat or animal products is not the only way to get protein in your diet. While meat can be a good source of protein, some meats – especially the highly processed kind – can also lead to inflammation and other chronic issues[2]. Keep things interesting, try to incorporate as many different protein sources as you can. See below for some dietary protein source ideas.

Protein Sources:
- Meats/poultry: eggs, chicken, turkey, duck, lamb, beef, pork
- Fish/Seafood: Mackerel, salmon, trout, tuna*
- Nuts, seeds and nut butters: almond, cashew, walnut, pistachio, chia, Brazil nut, pumpkin seeds
- Legumes: lentils, kidney beans, black beans, chickpeas, pinto beans, lima beans, edamame
- Pay careful attention to the sourcing of your meat and seafood. How was it raised? Were hormones or antibiotics involved? Was the animal healthy? If you are getting your meat from a local butcher, these are great questions to ask. If you are getting your meat from a grocery store, the farm is usually listed on the label. Do some research to learn more

about where your meat is coming from. Chances are if the animal was not raised in a sustainable, healthy manner, it is probably not a sustainable, healthy form of nutrition.

Day 3: Fruits and veggies

This is an important one. I might argue that it is even more important than protein. Fruits and vegetables are high in those micronutrients we were talking about yesterday. They are full of vitamins and minerals as well as constituents like flavonoids and antioxidants that can help lower inflammation-[3]. If you are someone who experiences chronic pain, you may have heard that lowering inflammation can help with reducing pain. Regularly eating adequate amounts of fruits and vegetables can help with managing pain over time by addressing inflammation.

> Question: What fruits and vegetables should you eat?
>
> Answer: As many different ones as you can!

The more colourful your diet, the better. Get creative and try to make at least half your plate fruits and vegetables.

Today's task is to try a fruit or vegetable that you have never tried before. Go to your usual grocery store, local farmer's market, backyard garden, or order online. Go wherever you usually get your produce from or venture somewhere new, choose a new fruit or vegetable, find out how to eat it and write about your experience. If you are feeling extra creative, look up some recipes and try them out. Maybe even invite someone to try the new discovery with you.

> **Wisdom Bite 5**: Juices are a treat! Yes, they have the same great micronutrients that you would find in the fruits and veggies that were used to make them,

but they also have all of the sugar and not much fiber. Be wary of too much juice.

Wisdom Bite 6: Fruits are higher in sugar than vegetables so if you already have larger amounts of sugar in your diet, try to aim for more vegetables than fruits.

Wisdom Bite 7: Variety in the diet is important. If you find yourself always eating the same foods, you may want to ask your Naturopathic Doctor about potential food sensitivities.

Day 4: Grains, breads, and starches

The typical North American diet includes a lot of grains, breads, and starches. These foods are very high in carbohydrates, a macronutrient. Simple carbohydrates are quickly converted into sugars for our body to use for energy, which can be useful especially if you are someone who has trouble gaining weight. However, with there being so much sugar available to us these days, this is probably a category you want to eat with cautious moderation.

    Some examples of foods in this category are bread/toast, pasta, rice, potatoes, quinoa, oats, millet, barley, corn.

    A really great time to eat foods that are high in simple carbohydrates would be right before exercising. They can quickly give your body some fuel to help you get through the work-out.

    Today's task is to try to have carbohydrates take up less than one third of your plate for every meal today.

Day 5: Healthy fats

Fats are important macronutrients too! They are important for brain health, the nervous system, heart and liver health. They also help with absorption of fat-soluble vitamins like Vitamins A, D, E, and K. It is important to note, however, that not all fats are the same.

There are saturated fats like those found in milk, some vegetable oils, butter, and animal products. These are the fats that have been associated with chronic heart disease[4].

There are unsaturated fats which include things like olive oil and fish oil. These are the fats that have been linked with lower risk of heart disease[5].

There is also cholesterol which is required for proper cell structure and function, brain and nervous system development, and hormone production.

There are many great ways to get more of these foods into your diet. Try adding olive oil to your salad, snacking on nuts or seeds, eating more fish or even try making your own guacamole.

Today's challenge is to see how many ways you can sneak healthy fats into your diet.

> **Wisdom Bite 8**: Heating oils over high heat, like frying them, changes their structure and may affect their nutrient value and taste. Try adding them to the end of a stir fry as opposed to cooking your food in the oil. If you are heating oils, opt for ones that have a higher smoke point.

Day 6: Whole foods for whole bodies

When I'm referencing whole foods, I am usually referring to a food that came from nature and has not been changed too much. That is, it has not been mixed with other ingredients like preservatives, sugar, or chemicals made in a lab. A whole food probably does not have an ingredient list attached to it. My view of whole foods includes things like fresh, dried, or frozen fruits and vegetables, grains, and minimally processed meat, fish and eggs.

However, with processed foods being so abundantly available in grocery stores and seemingly so convenient, it can sometimes be a little too easy to reach for the ready-to-eat, processed foods over the whole foods that we then have to prepare. I am very much a strong advocate for preparing your own food and there is research to show that preparing your own food is linked to positive diet changes and more cooking confidence[6]. That being said, I can also understand that some days, it is easier or seems to make more sense to reach for the convenient options.

If you are going to purchase a prepared or processed food, read the ingredients first. Educate yourself on what you are putting in your body. Paying careful attention to ingredients you simply do not recognize can be an opportunity to learn more about these ingredients. Also pay attention to sugar content. It can be surprising to see how many products sugar finds its way into.

Today's task: For the next 24 hours, pay attention to how many whole foods you are eating and journal it. Remember, we are defining a whole food as anything that came from nature like fruits, vegetables, grains, or animals, has not been unrecognizably changed from its original form, and does not have an ingredient list associated with it.

Day 7: The grocery shop

What a week! It is time to put everything we learned about nutrition this week together.

Today's task is to plan your next trip to the grocery store.

The first step is to take a look at the food journal you started at the beginning of the week. After all the learning you have done this week, are there any changes you would like to make?

The next step is to make a list; what would you like to try adding to your diet, are there any new recipes you would like to try? If this seems overwhelming reach out to your Naturopathic Doctor, holistic nutritionist, dietician or health coach for help.

Some helpful resources and tips for planning your grocery shop:

1. Look into food boxes, food shares, or food ordering services for some healthy convenient options.
2. Find out about local farmer's markets or cooperative grocery stores in your area. This can also be a great way to get to know your neighbours and foster a sense of community.
3. Head to your local grocery store and spend the most time in the outer aisles of the store. Did you know that most grocery stores are organized to have their fresh foods and produce on the outer edges of the store and their processed foods in the middle aisles of the store? It is important to note however that there are still some gems in the grocery store aisles like dried beans, herbal teas and spices.

Wisdom Bite 9: Dried, frozen, and canned fruits and vegetables can also be wonderfully nutritious affordable options, especially during the winter months in Canada when many of them are not in season or not available locally.

Wisdom Bite 10: Try organizing your pantry or fridge to make the food that you have clearly visible. This can help with prepping meals, using what you have, and preventing food waste.

A note on supplements: Supplements can be a great way to get extra nutrients in that might be missing from the diet. Talk to your Naturopathic Doctor or other knowledgeable health professional about which supplements may be helpful for you.

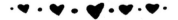

A breath of fresh air: Did you know that what you eat affects how you breathe? For example, the body's breakdown of carbohydrates produces more carbon dioxide than the breakdown of fats which may require you to breathe harder to eliminate it[7]. On the other hand, how you breathe can affect your nutrition too! A few mindful breaths before a meal can help your body relax so that it can focus on properly digesting the meal.

---

1. Carbone JW, Pasiakos SM. Dietary Protein and Muscle Mass: Translating Science to Application and Health Benefit. Vol. 11, Nutrients . 2019.
2. Micha R, Wallace SK, Mozaffarian D. Epidemiology and Prevention Red and Processed Meat Consumption and Risk of Incident Coronary Heart Disease , Stroke , and Diabetes Mellitus A Systematic Review and Meta-Analysis. 2010
3. Holt EM, Steffen LM, Moran A, Basu S, Steinberger J, Ross JA, et al. Fruit and vegetable consumption and its relation to markers of inflammation and oxidative stress in adolescents. J Am Diet Assoc. 2009 Mar;109(3):414–21
4. National Research Council (US) Committee on Diet and Health. Diet and Health: Implications for Reducing Chronic Disease Risk. Washington (DC): National Academies Press (US); 1989. 7, Fats and Other Lipids. Available from: https://www.ncbi.nlm.nih.gov/books/NBK218759/
5. National Research Council (US) Committee on Diet and Health. Diet and Health: Implications for Reducing Chronic Disease Risk. Washington (DC): National Academies Press (US); 1989. 7, Fats and Other Lipids. Available from: https://www.ncbi.nlm.nih.gov/books/NBK218759/
6. Reicks M, Kocher M, Reeder J. Impact of Cooking and Home Food Preparation Interventions Among Adults: A Systematic Review (2011-2016). J Nutr Educ Behav. 2018 Feb;50(2):148–172 .e1.
7. Berthon BS, Wood LG. Nutrition and respiratory health--feature review. Nutrients. 2015 Mar 5;7(3):1618-43. doi: 10.3390/nu7031618. PMID: 25751820; PMCID: PMC4377870.

	Sunday	Monday	Tuesday	Wednesday	Thursday	Friday	Saturday
Breakfast							
AM snack							
Lunch							
PM snack							
Dinner							
Notes							

Exercise

Wahoo! You made it to the halfway point. You deserve a pat on the back.

This week we are talking about exercise and as I have mentioned at the beginning of every week, enjoyment is a key motivator so it should come as no surprise at this point when I say, the best exercise is fun exercise that brings you joy!

I also think that it is important to mention that movement looks different for everyone and that is okay. Recall our discussion on the myth of normal? Revisit week 1 if you need to jog your memory.

The purpose of this week will be to connect with your body through movement. Hopefully by the end of this week you will have a better understanding of your body, movement and how to keep moving. This may also be a good point to enlist the help of a physiotherapist, registered kinesiologist, or experienced personal trainer to guide you in this process. Check out our list of practitioners for some ideas.

Please note that this week, like the nutrition week, is a full one. You may find it helpful to space things out over two weeks. Listen to your body and be kind and gentle with yourself.

Day 1: **Range of motion**

When we talk about range of motion here, we are referring to the amount of movement you have at each joint.

There are two ways we can look at range of motion. There is **active** range of motion and **passive** range of motion. Active range of motion refers to the movement you can achieve on your own, using your muscles at each joint. Passive range of motion refers to the amount of movement you have around a joint without having to actively engage your muscles. Passive range of motion is best assessed when someone else is helping you to move your joints to see how much they can move.

Today we are going to figure out what your range of motion is at each of the major joints. I highly suggest you follow along with our YouTube video *One Month to Neuromuscular Health: Range of Motion*. Following along will significantly help you visualize how to safely move your joints through their ranges. Remember, we all move differently! This exercise is meant for you to understand how YOU move, let's approach this with curiosity, no need for comparison or judgment here.

Okay, how about we begin with active range of motion? Start in a position that feels comfortable for you; it can be standing, sitting, or even laying down.

Start with the head and neck. Nod your head up and down and turn your head side to side. How far can you go without any pain or discomfort?

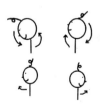

Next move to the shoulders. Shrug your shoulders up and down. Try seeing if you can make circles with your arms straight. Try moving your arms in forward circles and backward circles. How big can you make your circles? If you are lying down, try moving your arms up and down like you are making a snow angel.

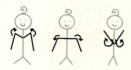

Time for the elbows. See if you can touch your shoulders, then straighten your arms again. Can you make it all the way to shoulders? Can you fully straighten your arms?

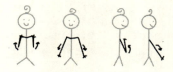

On to the wrists. See if you can make little circles with your wrists. How big are these circles? Try going both clockwise and counter-clockwise. Do you notice any differences between the two movements? How about any differences between the right and left wrists?

Time for the fingers. Try making your hands into fists and then opening them and spreading out your fingers. Try this movement a couple of times. How does it feel?

Now on to the hips. If you're standing, try making big circles with your hips as if trying to keep a hula hoop up. How big can you make the circles? If you're sitting or lying down, try bringing your knees to your chest one at a time, how far can you go?

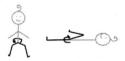

Time for the knees! If you're standing, try standing on one leg and bringing your heel to your behind. Then try straightening your legs, one at a time. Can your heel make it all the way to your bum? If you are sitting, try straightening and bending your legs one at a time. How straight can you get your legs without leaning backward? If you are laying down, you may have to involve your hips a little bit. Bring your knees to a bent position, then try straightening them, one at a time. Remember the laying down position involves both the hips and knees so may be a little harder than the seated and standing positions.

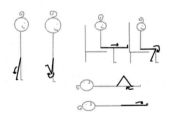

Ankle time. Just like you did with the wrists, try making little circles with your ankles. How big are the circles? Any differences in your ankles versus your wrists?

Finally, we're down to your toes. Try bending and straightening your toes. How much movement can you get there?

And we did it! We went through the whole body, head to toe. Take some time to thank your body for the movement you just did no matter how big or small. Take some time to also reflect on how you are feeling physically, mentally, and emotionally after this exercise.

Day 2: Stretch it out

The importance of stretching cannot be overstated. This is a key activity when it comes to neuromuscular health. There are so many ways to stretch too! This week, we are going to focus on two types of simple stretching techniques but as we discussed in week one, enjoyment is paramount so I encourage you to find a stretching routine that you enjoy.

Today we are going to focus on **dynamic stretching**. Dynamic stretching involves moving stretches as opposed to stretches that are more like poses and held for longer periods of time. I find dynamic stretching to be quite fun! These stretches are also great to do before strength training because they can help reduce muscle stiffness and increase the range of motion around joints[1]. You probably remember what range of motion is from yesterday's activity and we will talk about strength training a little later on this week.

Today's activity is quite simple as it builds on yesterday's. In fact, you already did some dynamic stretching yesterday! Today we are simply repeating yesterday's exercise by taking each joint through its full range of motion, except this time we are going to do the exercise three times for each joint. Remember to check out the YouTube video *One Month to Neuromuscular Health: Range of Motion* for demonstrations.

Day 3: Really stretch it out

If you have been working on this program daily, you have now stretched two days in a row... congratulations! Have you noticed any differences in your movement or how you are feeling? Journal it, even if the answer is no.

Today we are going to be working on **static stretching**. This type of stretching involves stretches that are held for about 30 seconds at a time and is best done after strength training or before bed.

Today we will be doing a full body stretch. The activity below will take you through stretching some of the major muscles of the body. Check out our Youtube video *One Month to*

Neuromuscular Health: Static Stretching for some demonstrations. Also note that while most of our attention today will be focused on feeling the stretch in the muscles, you may also notice you feel some soreness or tiredness in opposing muscles since we may be using those to help with stretching.

Neck
1. Tuck your chin to your chest and imagine a string at the top of your head pulling it upward. Hold for 30 seconds. You should feel this stretch at the back of your neck.
2. Look up toward the sky. Hold for 30 seconds. You should feel this stretch at the front of your neck. If you notice any pain or discomfort at the back of your neck, skip this stretch.
3. Looking straight ahead, try touching your left ear to your left shoulder. You should feel this stretch on the right side of your neck. Hold for 30 seconds.
4. Looking straight ahead, try touching your right ear to your right shoulder. You should feel this stretch on the left side of your neck. Hold for 30 seconds.

Shoulders
1. Keeping your shoulders back and down, raise both arms to the sides as high as they will go. Hold for 30 seconds. You should feel this stretch in your chest and under your arms or in your triceps muscles.
2. Keeping your shoulders back and down, raise both arms forward as high as they will go. Hold for 30 seconds. You should feel this stretch under your arms.

Back
1. Give yourself a hug and curl forward like a cat arching it's back. Hold for 30 seconds. You should feel this stretch between your shoulder blades.

Chest
1. With your arms down by your sides and palms facing forward, raise your arms to the side as you squeeze your shoulder blades together and push your chest forward. Hold for 30 seconds. You should feel this stretch through the front of your chest or pectoral muscles. To increase the stretch,

with palms still facing forward, bend elbows 90 degrees, remembering to keep shoulders back and down.

Abdomen
1. Clasp your hands together in front of you and raise your arms as high as you can. Shift as much of your weight as you can onto the front or balls of your feet. Hold for 30 seconds. You should feel this stretch through your abdomen and maybe even your hip flexors.

Legs
1. Keeping your back straight and hands on your hips, hinge forward from your hips. Imagine there is a string attached to your tailbone, pulling it up toward the sky. Hold for 30 seconds. You should feel this stretch behind your legs or in your hamstring muscles. If you are feeling any lower back pain, try bending your knees slightly.
2. Use the back of a chair or table for balance if needed for this one. Bring your left heel to your left butt cheek. Hold for 30 seconds. You should feel this stretch through the top front of your left leg or quadriceps muscle.
3. Again, use the back of a chair or table for balance if needed. Bring your right heel to your right butt cheek. Hold for 30 seconds. You should feel this stretch through the top front of your right leg or quadriceps muscle.
4. While seated on a chair, with your legs dangling or extended straight out in front of you, flex your toes toward you and push your heels away. Hold for 30 seconds. You should feel this stretch in the back of your lower legs or gastrocnemius muscles.

Day 4: Building strength

Today we are going to be talking about strength training, which is all about making our muscles stronger. Before we get into some exercises, it is important to remember the importance of nutrition when it comes to increasing muscle mass. In order to build muscle, we need to have the right fuel.

Carbohydrates and fats can help give us energy for our work-out and protein can help with muscle repair. Do you recall last week when we talked about protein helping with building muscle? I generally like to have a quick snack that is higher in carbohydrates before starting strength training (like a banana with almond butter) and a larger snack or meal after strength-training that is higher in protein. If you need to, look back on last week's nutrition notes to jog your memory. There are also many supplements and even botanical medicines than can help with improving endurance, energy, and building muscle. For example, there is a significant amount of research on creatine supplementation and improving muscle strength[2] [3]. I would suggest working with a Naturopathic Doctor or other knowledgeable healthcare provider to learn more about these, which ones would be helpful for you, and how to incorporate them into your daily routine.

Now on to exercise! Strength training involves using your muscles to push against some sort of resistance, whether it is a resistance band, weights, your own body weight, or even gravity. The key to strength training is to start where you are right now and make slow and steady gains over time. Maybe today you are starting with moving your muscles without resistance. When that gets too easy, you can add some resistance. When that gets too easy, you can increase the resistance. It is helpful to track your progress over time.

Today we are going to start with a simple strength training exercise: the classic push-up. I'm going to remind you here, yet again, how important it is to remember that everyone is different and everyone moves differently. This means that the classic push-up will look different for everyone. I will outline some push-up variations below. Start with the one that feels challenging for you but is not sore or painful. It is important to listen to your body here as pushing it too hard can result in injury. Over time you can progress to the more challenging versions as you get stronger. Please follow along with our Youtube video *One Month to Neuromuscular Health: The Push Up* where Jalee and I demonstrate how to safely do these variations.

Seated Push-up
Starting with your elbows against your sides, arms bent and palms facing outward, straighten your arms as if you are pushing something really heavy away from you. Bring your arms back and repeat this motion 10 times. Really visualize pushing the heavy thing away from you, you should feel this in your biceps and triceps muscles. Take a 30 second break, then repeat for another two sets of 10.

Seated Push-up against a resistance band
Stretch a resistance band across your mid-back and hold each end of the band in each hand. Starting with your elbows against your sides, arms bent and palms facing outward, straighten your arms forward against the resistance band. Bring your arms back and repeat this motion 10 times. You should feel this in your biceps and triceps muscles. Take a 30 second break, then repeat for another two sets of 10.

Standing push-up against a table
Form a diagonal line with your body against the table so that your arms are straight out in front of you, hands are on the edge of the table, your chest is over the edge of the table, your back and legs are straight in a plank position with feet on the floor. Bend your elbows to bring your chest to the table, then straighten your arms again. Be sure to keep your elbows tucked to your sides and repeat the movement 10 times. You should feel this in your biceps and triceps muscles. Take a 30 second break, then repeat for another two sets of 10.

Standing push-up against a wall
Stand parallel to a wall with arms straight out in front of you and hands on the wall. Bend your elbows to bring your chest to the wall, then straighten your arms again. Be sure to keep elbows tucked to your sides and repeat the movement 10 times. You should feel this in your biceps and triceps muscles. Take a 30 second break, then repeat for another two sets of 10.

Push-up on knees
On your hands and knees on the floor, with arms straight, and elbows tucked in toward your sides, lower yourself down to

the floor, then push yourself back up. Repeat the movement 10 times. You should feel this in your biceps and triceps muscles. Take a 30 second break, then repeat for another two sets of 10.

Push up against the floor
Start in a plank position so that your back and legs are straight, toes are touching the floor, arms are stretched out in front of you with hands on the floor. Lower yourself down to the floor, then push yourself back up. Be sure to keep elbows tucked to your sides and repeat the movement 10 times. You should feel this in your biceps and triceps muscles. Take a 30 second break, then repeat for another two sets of 10.

> **A note on intention**: As you will see at the end of next week, visualization and intention is key when it comes to building strength. In fact, simply **imagining** moving a muscle without actually moving the muscle can increase the strength of that muscle[4]! Stay tuned for more details on the study that demonstrated this interesting phenomenon next week when we work on bringing our intentions to life.

Day 5: Sweat it out

Let's talk about the heart. This is a very important muscle that helps deliver nutrients to all of your other muscles. The heart is a muscle that never really rests and pumps day in and day out. Before we get into today's exercise for the heart, take a minute to thank your heart for all its hard work.

Now that we have thanked our hard-working heart, let's get into cardiorespiratory exercise, also known as cardio. The idea of cardio is something that has made me cringe in the past because of the expectations I had around what it needed to look like. However, like all the exercise we have talked about so far, exercise for your heart and lungs can also be enjoyable!

There are all the classic forms of cardio like running, jogging, walking, biking etc. but there are also ones that you may not have considered to be cardio. For example: dancing, swimming, hiking, foraging through the forest (one of my personal favourites), and gardening are all examples of cardio. Even kissing a significant other can give your heart a little work-out.

Today's task is to try an activity that gets your heart beating a little faster. To start we are going to measure our resting heart rate. This is how fast our heart beats while we are at rest. If you have a fancy watch or other technology to measure your heart rate, you may be familiar with this. However, today we are going to measure our heart rate the old fashioned way.

First, find your pulse. The easiest place to find it is on the side of your neck. You can find it by using your index and middle fingers to feel the area right next to where you might find an Adam's apple. Keep feeling around until you can feel your heart beat. This is your carotid pulse.

Pull out a timer and set it to 60 seconds. Count how many times your heart beats during that time. This is your pulse. The average pulse at rest ranges from 60-100 beats per minute (bpm). What is yours?

Now that you have your resting heart rate, let's do some cardio and get that heart beating a little faster. Ideally, you want to increase your heart rate and feel your breathing get a little faster.

For example, you could try doing jumping jacks, punching the air (or a punching bag), or running on the spot until you start to feel short of breath but are still able to carry a conversation if you needed to.

Now measure your pulse again. What is it now? Has it changed?

Day 6: How do you like to move?

In case it hasn't sunk in yet, enjoying exercise is so important! Who wants to spend time doing something they do not enjoy?

Today you are going to brainstorm some activities that you find enjoyable. To do this we are going to first connect with what joy feels like for you. Take a moment to close your eyes and picture the last time you felt joyful or happy. What were you doing? Who were you with? What did it feel like? What did you feel in your body? What thoughts did you have? Were there any smells or tastes?

Now, in your journal, make a list of activities that bring that sense of joy.

Do any of these activities involve stretching, strength training, cardio or all three? For example, I love gardening and it involves all three! I also love tai chi and qigong which involves stretching and strengthening.

Highlight the activities that involve stretching, circle the ones that involve strength training, underline the ones that involve cardio, and draw a box around the ones that involve all three.

Day 7: Putting it all together

We have talked at length about the importance of enjoying exercise. Now, we are going to talk about the importance of consistency. Consistency is paramount when it comes to any exercise. Think of taking care of a plant. Plants need care on a regular basis. If you only water your plant every couple of months when you notice it is dried out and dying, your plant is probably not going to do very well. However, if you check on your plant every day, remove dead leaves or flowers, trim it every so often, water it as needed, and treat it with loving kindness your plant will probably do quite well. The same goes for you and your muscles. If you move your muscles every day, it will be a lot easier to keep them moving than if you only decide to stretch the week before that check in with your doctor or when you are feeling stiff and in pain.

Today we are going to bring everything from this week together to come up with a plan to incorporate regular movement into your daily life.

Let's start with stretching. Dynamic and static stretching like we demonstrated in days 2 and 3 this week can be done every day, at any time of day, and as many times in the day as you wish. You can do the stretching exercises we did together earlier this week or even one of the stretching activities you listed yesterday.

I like starting and ending my day with a good stretch or adding some stretching in after lunch on a busy day.

Strength training can get a little trickier. Here you want to make sure that you are listening to your body and balancing exercise with rest and recovery. Start small and work your way up as you get more comfortable. It might look something like starting with a five- to ten-minute strength training activity once per week. When you feel like you have mastered that, add in a second activity, ensuring rest days in between. When you have mastered that, try increasing the duration of the activities by five or ten minutes. Keep working your way up in this fashion until you feel satisfied with your weekly activities.

If you have not done so already, this would be a very good time to enlist a physiotherapist or kinesiologist to help you come up with a safe and effective plan for incorporating strength training into your daily routine.

When it comes to cardio, the Heart and Stroke Foundation of Canada recommends 150 minutes per week in bouts of ten minutes at a time[5]. If ten minutes at a time seems like too much, start with five minutes and work your way up. Remember, if you are doing a cardio activity that you enjoy, it may be easier to keep it up for longer.

Today's task is to schedule in some movement this week. Schedule at least one or two stretching activities per day, one or two cardio activities per day, and at least one strength training activity in the week. I like planning my movement weekly and like taking Sundays off with no scheduled activity. Find a system that works for you!

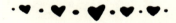

A breath of fresh air: Did you know mindful breathing can play an important role in exercise? Start with paying attention to your breathing while you are moving. Are you holding your breath? Are you breathing faster or slower? As you become more aware of your breathing you can start to link it to your movement. For example, taking a breath in while you stretch and breathing out when you relax.

1. Opplert J, Babault N. Acute Effects of Dynamic Stretching on Muscle Flexibility and Performance: An Analysis of the Current Literature. Sports Med. 2018 Feb;48(2):299–325.
2. Kley RA, Tarnopolsky MA, Vorgerd M. Creatine for treating muscle disorders. Cochrane Database Syst Rev [Internet]. 2013;(6). Available from: https://doi.org//10.1002/14651858.CD004760.pub4
3. Wax B, Kerksick CM, Jagim AR, Mayo JJ, Lyons BC, Kreider RB. Creatine for Exercise and Sports Performance, with Recovery Considerations for Healthy Populations. Nutrients. 2021 Jun;13(6).
4. Ranganathan VK, Siemionow V, Liu JZ, Sahgal V, Yue GH. From mental power to muscle power--gaining strength by using the mind. Neuropsychologia. 2004;42(7):944–56.
5. Heart and Stroke Foundation of Canada. How much physical activity do you need? [Internet]. Health Seekers. 2021. Available from: https://www.heartandstroke.ca/healthy-living/stay-active/how-much-physical-activity-do-you-need

Connection

Congratulations! You have made it to the last week!
  Hopefully you are starting to feel empowered about your health, especially when it comes to your neuromuscular health. In the last three weeks of the course, we have spent a lot of time looking at you, how you feel, changes you can make, etc.
  This week we are going to expand your bubble and start looking at the people around you, who you connect with, and support networks. Community and a sense of belonging is a very important aspect of health. Feeling well-supported and connected to something bigger than yourself brings perspective and makes everything we have talked about so far become much easier to work through. In fact, it seems that feeling well-supported can help those living with chronic pain better adjust to and cope with their pain[1].

Day 1: Who's in your corner?

We all need help from time to time. Sometimes it can be hard to ask for help, but life becomes so much easier when we do. Have you ever noticed how good it feels to help someone out? When you ask for help, you may even be gifting someone with the opportunity to do something nice for you.

Today we are going to talk about the people in your support network. These are the people who you feel like you can lean on when you need some extra help.

The first step of today's task is to write a list of the people you would feel comfortable asking for help.

Some follow-up questions to ask yourself:
- How do you feel about your list?
- Are you grateful to have these people in your life?
- Is there room for improvement?
- Do you need to build a stronger support network? How can you do that?
- Do you struggle with asking for help?
- How often do you help others?

Day 2: Whose corner are you in?

We talked a little bit yesterday about how great it can feel to help someone out. Do you remember the last time you helped someone out? How did it feel?

Today we are going to take a look at the people who you support. Remember that support can come in so many different ways!

The first step of today's task is similar to yesterday's. Make a list of the people who you would feel comfortable offering help or support to.

How does today's list compare to yesterday's? You can even ask yourself the same follow-up questions. What do you notice about your answers?

Yesterday's follow-up questions:
- How do you feel about your list?
- Are you grateful to have these people in your life?
- Is there room for improvement?
- Do you need to build a stronger support network? How can you do that?
- Do you struggle with asking for help?
- How often do you help others?

CONNECTION

Day 3: Communities

Today we are going to take support networks a step further and take a look at which communities you are involved in. There are so many different types of communities. Some examples are: family, friend groups, book clubs, garden clubs, church groups, school classmates, work colleagues, support groups, etc.

Can you see where we are going with today's task? Today we are going to make a list of all of the communities that you are a part of. What do you like about being a part of these communities? How do you contribute to these communities? Do these communities bring you feelings of joy and connection?

Day 4: Connecting to something bigger

We spent the last three days talking about your connection to other people. Now it is time to expand that network to include nature, the universe, a higher being, your sense of purpose; whatever it is that you connect to that is bigger than you.

Take some time today to connect in a way that works for you.

If you are struggling with figuring out how to connect, I usually like to start with connecting with nature because this is something everyone can do. You are also welcome to pray or meditate if that is how you prefer to connect.

Here are some of my favourite ways to reconnect when I am feeling disconnected:
- Water my house plants
- Spend some time in the garden
- Invite a friend over for tea
- Go for a walk
- Spend some time in the forest
- Go to the beach
- Pray the rosary or use prayer beads
- Light a candle, play some music, and quietly connect with God
- Watch the snow fall
- Watch the rain fall
- Wake up to see the sunrise
- Head to the best spot to see the sun set

- Say a prayer of gratitude

Remember the plant metaphor we talked about last week when we were discussing the importance of consistency? Taking time to connect is also something that is best done regularly. Don't wait until you feel disconnected, take some time to connect daily.

Day 5: Revisiting intentions

Now it's time to think all the way back to the end of week one when you set your intentions. Do you remember what they were? You should have them written down so take another look. After your month of working on neuromuscular health, do you feel like these intentions still make sense for you? Is there anything that you would like to change?

Write down your new intentions (or the same ones again if there isn't anything about them that you would like to change). Feel free to be creative or bring your artistic side out to decorate these intentions so that you are inspired to look at them. Place them somewhere visible and whenever you look at them, imagine what it will feel like when they are true.

Day 6: Bringing intentions to life

Now that we have our intentions written down and visible, it seems like a good time to do a visualization exercise to really feel what it will be like when they are true. Did you know visualization can be a really useful tool when it comes to bringing our intentions to life? In fact, a 2004 study found that people who only **imagined** moving their fingers and flexing their biceps actually increased their strength without physically moving their fingers or arms[2]. How cool is that? This is also really important to keep in mind when it comes to exercising, especially if there is an exercise you're not quite strong enough to do yet. Simply visualizing the movement you want to do may actually help in increasing the strength of the muscles required to complete the movement.

Let's get started on the visualization activity. Read through the whole activity first so you know what comes next after you close your eyes.

Visualization activity:

First get grounded, take some deep breaths in and out, sit or lie in a comfortable position and close your eyes. If it helps, you can even have soft music playing in the background.

Start with one intention at a time. Imagine that intention is already true.

What does it feel like?
Who are with?
What are you doing?
What is happening around you?
What does life look like?
What steps did you need to take to get there?

Day 7: Wrap-up

You made it! One month to neuromuscular health down, many more to go. Remember healing is always a journey. There are ups and downs and lots of learning along the way. Take some time today to reflect on your journey, congratulate yourself for making it to the end, and start on the next steps of your healing journey.

---

1. López-Martínez AE, Esteve-Zarazaga R, Ramírez-Maestre C. Perceived Social Support and Coping Responses Are Independent Variables Explaining Pain Adjustment Among Chronic Pain Patients. J Pain [Internet]. 2008;9(4):373–9. Available from: https://www.sciencedirect.com/science/article/pii/S1526590007010280
2. Ranganathan VK, Siemionow V, Liu JZ, Sahgal V, Yue GH. From mental power to muscle power--gaining strength by using the mind. Neuropsychologia. 2004;42(7):944–56.

Complimentary Care Resource Network - NMD

Name	Title	Credentials	Clinic Location	Phone Number	Email	Website	Accessibility
Felicia Assenza	Naturopathic Doctor	HBsc, ND	1601 King St. E Hamilton, ON L8K 1T5	905-544-5834	felicia.assenza@gmail.com	drfeliciaassenzand.com	clinic has 3 stairs (steps) to entrance virtual visits available
Felicia Assenza	Naturopathic Doctor	HBsc, ND	Awakening Health 4300 Upper Middle Rd. Unit 3 Burlington, ON L7M 4P6	905-335-0372	Felicia@awakeninghealth.ca	awakeninghealth.ca	Yes
Bridget Ross	Naturopathic Doctor	Bsc, ND	Virtual services available	416 738 8593	bridgetrossnd@gmail.com	bridgetrossnd.com	Yes (virtual)
Andy Schmalz	Osteopathic Practitioner	DO(MP), CAT(C)	Awakening Health 4300 Upper Middle Rd. Unit 3 Burlington, ON L7M 4P6	905-335-0372	admin@awakeninghealth.ca	awakeninghealth.ca	Yes
Angelika Baum	Belief Change and Relationship Coach		Awakening Health 4300 Upper Middle Rd. Unit 3 Burlington, ON L7M 4P6	905-335-0372	greendoorrelaxation@yahoo.ca	awakeninghealth.ca	Yes
Dan Bosy	Physiotherapist Myofascial release practitioner	BSc. (P.T.) Dip. Manip Fellow of CAMPT	Awakening Health 4300 Upper Middle Rd. Unit 3 Burlington, ON L7M 4P6	905-335-0372	Dan@awakeninghealth.ca	awakeninghealth.ca	Yes
Melissa Dermody	Physiotherapist (pediatrics and adults)	PT (MSc PT)	Paediatric Physiotherapy Associates, 3701 Danforth avenue (Variety Village location) Scarborough ON, M1N2G2	647-444-9219	melissadermody.pt@gmail.com	https://www.paediatricphysiotherapy.com/	Yes
Julie Bellini	Registered Kinesiologist	RK, OKA, CKO	High Performance Solutions Mobile (Virtual/Mobile)	905-961-0749	julie.hpsmobile@gmail.com	HPSmobile.ca	Yes (virtual)
Thomas Eagles	Registered Kinesiologist Osteopathic Manual Practitioner	BSc Kin, R. Kin. D.O.M.P, DSc.O	Freemotion Therapy 1233 Main St. E Hamilton, ON L8K 1A5	289-925-0445	info@freemotiontherapy.ca	freemotiontherapy.ca	Yes
Anita Verigin	Registered Massage Therapist	RMT	Freemotion Therapy 1233 Main St. E Hamilton, ON L8K 1A5	289-925-0445	info@freemotiontherapy.ca	freemotiontherapy.ca	Yes
Jacob Kang	Chiropractor	MSc, DC	Leaside Chiro and Scoliosis Centre 860 Millwood Road Toronto, ON M4G 1W6	647-347-7125	torontoscoliosiscentre@gmail.com	http://leasidechiro.com	
Dr. Phil DiFilippo	Chiropractor	HBScKin, DC	Rosedale Chiropractic Clinic 230 Graham Avenue S Hamilton, Ontario L7M 4V3	905-545-7570		rosedalechiropractic.ca	5 stairs (steps) to reception
Andrea Falco	Psychotherapist	M.Ed, RCC	Virtual, services available for British Columbia residents	647-448-1324	afalcocounselling@gmail.com	andreafalco.ca	Yes (Virtual)
Brooklyn Marx	Registered Psychotherapist (Qualifying)	BSc., MA, RP(Q)	Virtual, services available for Ontario residents	519-270-8233	brooklyn@raisingfamiliestherapy.com	raisingfamiliestherapy.com	Yes (virtual)

Acknowledgments

This book would not have been possible without the support of so many. A generous thank you to family, friends, and colleagues who supported the completion of this project, providing input and resources along the way. A special thank you to the incredible focus group who courageously tried the program first and helped ensure its efficacy and safety for those who try it next.

Author and Contributors

Author: Felicia Assenza, ND

Felicia is a Naturopathic Doctor whose own healthcare experiences lead her to discover the benefits of naturopathic medicine. She earned her Bachelor of Science degree at McMaster University in 2013, majoring in Biology & Psychology. Her interest in the mind and brain lead her to complete an Honours thesis in behavioural neuroscience, investigating emotional regulation and mood disorders in adolescents.

She then went on to earn her Doctor of Naturopathy degree at the Canadian College of Naturopathic Medicine in 2017. While there, she had the pleasure of interning on a pediatric-focused clinical shift, a clinical placement in the Queen West Community Health Centre in Toronto, Ontario. She also completed a global clinical preceptorship in Northern India.

Felicia aims to share knowledge and experiences gained on her own journey to help others on their health journeys. Gentle curiosity guides her practice and much time is spent in office visits exploring symptoms and making connections to discover their root cause. She also loves food and gardening and believes both are among the most powerful medicines.

Contributor: Jalee Pelissier, PTA, OTA

Jalee is a strong advocate for neuromuscular health. Her own experiences with a neuromuscular disorder drove her to start advocating for neuromuscular health at the young age of thirteen. Her advocacy work led her to become an honorary firefighter in her hometown of Sudbury, Ontario.

In 2020, Jalee completed her education at College Boreal as a Physiotherapy and Occupational Therapy Assistant and spent some time working in long-term care. Jalee also serves as a spokesperson for the Sunshine Foundation of Canada, sits on the Accessibility Advisory Panel of the City of Sudbury, and currently works for Muscular Dystrophy Canada.

Her knowledge and experience was invaluable in designing the exercise aspect of this program and her passion for neuromuscular health inspired the roots of this program.

Editor: Pauline Nichol, MRT(R)

Pauline Nichol is a Medical Radiation Technologist and the author of the poetry collection *A Break in the Clouds*. As both a healthcare provider and writer, Pauline's science and healthcare background combined with her artful literary expertise was an asset to completing the book you have before you.